WILL SOMEONE PLEASE SHOOT THE CUCKOO?

One woman's continuing journey through

hypothyroidism and today's healthcare system.

Also by the Author

Genealogy

Metes & Bound I: Dugal McQueen and Some Descendants
Metes & Bounds II: David Crews, Ancestors & Descendants
(1st Edition 1993, 2nd Edition 2014)
Metes & Bounds III: John McQueen & Nancy Crews, Children & Grandchildren

I Will Go With You: The Hechlers, Germany to Russia to America

Novels

Children of the Light Series
Keeping Secrets
Breaking Promises
Binding Fire

Front cover design: Donna Hechler Porter
Stock photography purchased with user license from 123rf.com. All photographs in author's personal collection.

Printed in the United States of America, First Printing, 2016
ISBN-13: 978-1539122067
ISBN-10: 1539122069

Dedicated to my grandmother

Robbie Eugene Griswold McQueen

May you now rest in peace . . .

WILL SOMEONE PLEASE

SHOOT THE CUCKOO?

One woman's continuing journey through

hypothyroidism and today's healthcare system

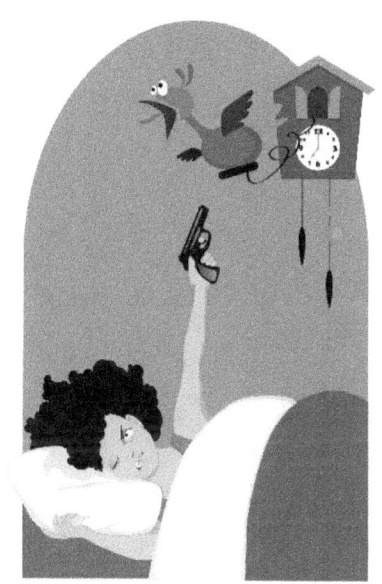

DONNA HECHLER
PORTER

INTRODUCTION

Did you pick this book up based on the title? Or perhaps it was the picture that caught your interest?

Cuckoo birds are annoying. The little beasts chirp and sing in the morning with a cheerful disposition while they fling their bodies outward over and over again.

Their message?

You are to rise and shine and meet another glorious day head on after a night of restful, rejuvenating sleep.

Or maybe not.

If you are a hypothyroid sufferer, it takes a long while and lots of work to wake with such enthusiasm in the morning. As a matter of fact, you may not be *waking* at all, but merely having been awake all night already, you simply drag yourself out of bed and try to cope with your day.

That's right – cope. Not live.

And yep – you are now beginning to understand my cover.

Untreated or poorly treated hypothyroid sufferers do not want to hear that blasted bird in the morning. They just want someone to take him away.

A great many others do not wish to face the morning at all. Some even feel as if they have become the cuckoo bird and are truly crazy – after all, no one believes them. Not family members, friends, and certainly not – gasp – most doctors.

Hypothyroidism is also a *silent* disease. Oftentimes people do not know we have it. The symptoms are vague and can come and go. We have no physical trappings or manifestations, especially in the early part of the disease. People will tell you all kinds of things – diet, exercise, take a walk, get out more. Family members, surprisingly, can be the most brutal of all.

People truly do not understand that all of those things are difficult for a hypothyroid sufferer even in the early stages.

In the later stages they can be impossible.

They do not understand our hatred of that bird, or clock, or whatever it is that wakes us in the morning to start a new day because, frankly, we have no steam to give the day.

Please note that this is not a book on thyroid disease and its clinical manifestations. I have included a quick overview of the thyroid gland and hypothyroidism in the Preface, and within the pages there is other information as it pertains to my own situation. I am a former schoolteacher turned writer, not a doctor nor a nurse. As such I have nothing in my background in regards to the medical profession besides my own road to health and doctoring my children, and I am not qualified beyond my own limited research to speak in depth of the medical aspects of this disease. There are a number of good books available for both scientific and medical information regarding hypothyroidism. If there are mistakes in presenting the information, they are all mine and no one else's.

What I can do is share with you my journey with this disease called hypothyroidism. It is a personal story fraught with pitfalls, setbacks, and sometimes steps forward and a return to normalcy, only to backslide again into ill health and that sometimes through no fault of my own.

And why do I wish to share my journey with you?

Because I believe that doctors do not know all the answers.

Because I talk to people all the time who have symptoms similar to mine who seem to get no help from their doctors, and/or they *doctor hop* in an effort to find a hero/heroine to fix their fuddled mind and battered body.

Because I believe that oftentimes disease is simply not as complicated as we are made to believe.

Because I believe we <u>must</u> be our own best advocate when it comes to our health.

Because I believe that hearing stories of any kind empowers people, and I hope to encourage you, if you are someone like me or you know someone like me, to put yourself on your own journey to better health and a better life.

As for the cuckoo?

Nothing is more frustrating than facing morning when you have had little to no sleep sometimes for weeks and months. The cuckoo represents not only the alarm clocks, but all those things we have to get up and tend. In reality, we really wish it would just all go away.

If you feel this way – take heart. I have felt it, too. No hypothyroid sufferer has not. This disease may be silent, but you are not alone. And you can, with proper medication and help, get better.

You can sleep. You can have energy to exercise.

You can face your mornings and your days.

You can get control of your life once again.

People frequently ask me about my thyroid condition. By now, after ten long years of this, it is almost impossible to tell them of my journey in a few sentences.

In an hour. A day . . .

I write this book for those of you who would like to pick my brain, or anyone's brain, and who are looking for a friendly ear and someone who might understand and offer some help. Some hope.

Believe me – you are not alone.

PREFACE

Hypothyroidism is a disease of the thyroid gland, specifically an *underactive* or, as I like to say in regards to mine, a *non-working* thyroid. Finding figures for the number of individuals affected is difficult. Countries with a deficiency of iodine in the diet have a much higher number of afflicted individuals than those that do not. The different kinds of thyroid diseases, even several different causes and types of hypothyroidism, are generally further broken down when discussing the numbers of those affected. It appears, however, that officially 1 to 2% of the population in the United States is affected by hypothyroidism, with women a greater number. Interestingly, it is not uncommon for a woman to have her first experience with hypothyroidism after the pregnancy and birth of a child.

And this number is likely too low. It does not take into account those individuals that are not seeking help for their fatigue and are therefore not aware their problem might be hypothyroidism. It does not take into account those individuals that live marginally on the edge of having a problem and somehow manage to cope with a condition that does not deteriorate into a full-blown state of disease. It certainly does not take into account those that suspect they have hypothyroidism, but their bloodwork appears fine, a doctor tells them it is not their thyroid, and they go off in search of another cause for their strange and varied symptoms.

Interestingly, the most common cause of hypothyroidism word-wide is too little iodine (thus the difficulty in coming up with a worldwide number that is accurate). Of course if you live in the western world, specifically the United States, this is not likely to be your problem. Other factors, thus, come into play.

In the vast majority of other cases hypothyroidism is the result of Hashimoto's thyroiditis. Initially, Hashimoto's causes hyperthyroidism or an overactive thyroid, but later the condition becomes hypothyroidism and results in an underactive or non-working thyroid. Other causes of hypothyroidism, although less common, are previous treatments with radioactive iodine, injury to the hypothalamus or the anterior pituitary gland, certain medications, a congenital issue at birth, or previous thyroid surgery, such as removal of such due to cancer.

In some instances, as in mine, the cause is never known.

The thyroid gland itself is found in the front of the neck below the Adam's apple. It consists of two connected lobes and is shaped similar to a butterfly with an *isthmus,* or center that holds the two lobes together. The gland secretes thyroid hormones which influence a wide range of behaviors in the body, including metabolism, cardiovascular health, protein synthesis, and growth and development. Interestingly, the gland is larger in women than in men, and in pregnancy it increases in size.

This hormonal output is regulated by the *thyroid stimulating hormone,* or TSH, which is secreted from the anterior pituitary. This in turn is regulated by thyrotropin-releasing hormone, or TRH, which is produced by the hypothalamus.

The thyroid gland is an endocrine gland, and hypothyroidism is technically an endocrine disorder. Other such disorders are hyperthyroidism, Cushing's Syndrome, thyroid nodules, pituitary disorders and tumors, acromegaly, hypoparathyroidism, and on and on. As for hypothyroidism, it occurs when the thyroid gland produces insufficient thyroid hormones. By contrast, hyperthyroidism is a result of the thyroid over producing thyroid hormones. A number of symptoms accompany hypothyroidism: fatigue, weight gain, poor memory and concentration, loss of hair (particularly in a round patch just at the crown), shortness of breath, sore muscles, arthritis like symptoms, and on and on. The best complete list of symptoms can be found at www.stopthethyroidmadness.com.

As stated earlier, the primary function of the thyroid is the production of the hormones, in this case triiodothyronine (referred to as T3), thyroxine (known as T4), and peptide hormone calcitonin. A healthy thyroid gland secretes thyroxine (T4), which is in turn converted to triiodothyronine (T3) in other organs, including the liver. T3 binds to the thyroid hormone receptor which is present in the nucleus of cells. While here, it turns on particular genes and jumpstarts the production of specific proteins. Additionally, the hormone binds itself to the cell membrane which in turn affects such processes as the formation of blood vessels and cell growth. All of these processes within the thyroid are controlled by the thyroid stimulating hormone (TSH) which is secreted by the pituitary.

Obviously, these thyroid hormones are an integral part of the body system and they are driven and kept in balance between the hypothalamus – pituitary – and thyroid. When one of these fails, the others pitch in to compensate and the balanced production of hormones is thrown off.

This was certainly true in my case.

TABLE OF CONTENTS

THE LITTLE BLACK RAIN CLOUD HOVERS

I'm just a little black rain cloud,
Hovering under the honey tree.

Winnie-the-Pooh
A. A. Milne, *The Many Adventures of Winnie-the-Pooh*

The fall of 2005 found me going back to work for a second year at a local private school. The year before, I have to admit, had been a bit of a train wreck. I missed roughly twenty-one days largely due to one of the twins, who at the time were in kindergarten, being sick. Added to this was the usual stress involved in any mother going back to work or working in general.

Trying to prepare decent lunches for children with various allergies.

Trying to put a square meal on the table at supper time.

Trying to get homework done in the evening.

Trying to see that children still participated in all their activities like baseball, gymnastics, piano lessons, and church activities.

Trying to get lesson plans prepared.

Trying to get papers graded.

Trying to keep my sanity at home and at school.

Trying to do laundry.

Trying to grocery shop.

Trying to get enough sleep.

Trying to get enough sleep.

Trying to get enough sleep.

I used the word *trying*, because I was not really getting any of it done with any sort of gusto or quality the first year. I certainly was not as the second year rolled along.

Also, I meant *trying* three times in regards to sleep as well, for it was *truly* a work to try to get enough.

Sleep, for me, has always been problematic. Before my marriage, in my late twenties and early thirties, I would oftentimes get nearly ten hours plus, sometimes going to bed as early as 7:30 and getting up the next morning at 5:30 or 6:00 to get to work as an elementary teacher. As anyone knows who teaches, especially in the primary grades, from the time your feet hit the pavement in the parking lot your body does not slow down. (Your brain had better not either or someone may die.) Teachers get no breaks. They have to *run* to the bathroom when an opportunity presents itself (and sometimes when it does not). They *might* get about ten minutes to eat lunch without their students. The work is exhausting, and there is really no opportunity for pacing oneself during the day. I am not saying teaching is the **only** job like this by the way, but I do believe it is one of the worst.

For someone who had always needed a lot of sleep anyway, my body literally needed ten or more hours to function at this level of on-going, non-stop physical and mental activity. Anything less for too long simply left me sleepy and tired at best, unproductive and near dangerous at worst. In fact, this sleep problem had begun in my high school years, when I rarely got enough sleep due to band, twirling, and other activities as well as academics. I remember fighting sleep in my early morning classes. The only three things I remember about one particular world history class my junior or senior year was 1) the teacher was right out of college and very young and more interested in flirting with the boys than in teaching, 2) I knew more than she did, and 3) I spent most of my time trying to pry my eyes open so I could at least stay awake. This was not the only class I suffered through, but it is one that stands out in my memory. However, as most teens find themselves sleepy, little thought was given to my fatigue. Most teens also work themselves loose of this need by their early twenties. I, it appeared, never did.

I was lucky, though, that in my mid- to late 20s I could not only find the time to sleep that much, but I did usually sleep that much. When I got married, however, sleep became more elusive simply because of the demands of a house and a family, even if it was only one other person. When the twins came along, well, it was nothing short of a train wreck.

The year I went back to work I also had an added concern to the need for sleep, one which I did not talk to people of at the time. For years I had suffered from volleying bouts of chronic constipation and frequent bowel movements. This had started in my late 20s, but had gotten worse over the years.

My condition was more than likely genetic in nature. My great-grandmother Lily Corinne Gray Griswold died at the age of 61 after a month long bout of peritonitis, an abdominal infection caused by a perforation (leakage or a hole in) the intestines. Adding to her condition, but not a direct cause of her death, was a severe rectocele which she had suffered with for twenty years – since about the age of 41.

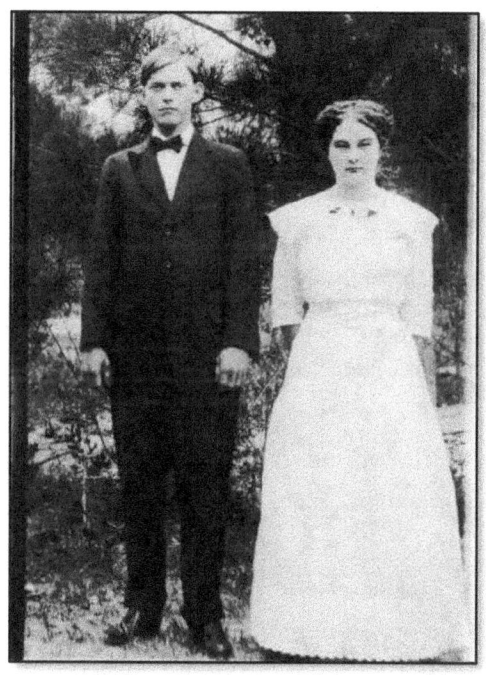

Charles Griswold & Lily Corinne Gray,
Wedding Picture, 1911, Polk County, Texas

Mama Lily, as she was known in later years, was born on 6 February 1895 in Louisiana to Alexander Gray and Huberta Kelley, daughter of Matthew Kelley and Sarah Honeycutt. Her mother had previously been married to Solomon Murray, and by him she had at least two living children by the 1880 census. Huberta married Alexander Gray, in 1890 after the death of Solomon. This was Alexander's first marriage.

About 1900 Alexander Gray decided to leave Louisiana for Texas, and Lily's mother supposedly died enroute as a result of childbirth. From stories Lily herself told, it sounded as if Huberta hemorrhaged either while pregnant or after the birth of this last child. I have been unable to locate the Grays in the 1900 census, so it is possible this was about the time they moved. Lily was about five or a bit older when her mother died. Huberta was in her early 40s at the time of her death. Alexander Gray remarried soon after to a woman named Katie Williamson.

Interestingly, Huberta's mother, Sarah Honeycutt Kelley (wife of Matthew Kelley), also died after Huberta's birth in 1856. Sarah was just past the age of 40, as was Huberta at the time of her death, and she too had given birth to at least four living children by this point, the last being Huberta herself. Yes, the similarities are rather eerie to say the least.

Of course childbirth in those days was a tricky thing. Women welcomed children even as they oftentimes feared the birthing process. Some women birthed a number of children, even upwards of ten or more even, never had much trouble, and later outlived their husbands. Other women were plagued with long, hard deliveries, perhaps gave birth to one or two children, and then subsequently died in a third or fourth pregnancy or birthing. More often than not, these tragic situations traveled in family groups, with a number of sisters, daughters and cousins, oftentimes dying after only one or two births. Genetics, it must be remembered, is a powerful force, and some women are just not born with the tissue strength of others.

How much of Lily's condition was shared by her mother and her grandmother in regards to childbirth and rectoceles is not known, and of course hemorrhaging, as in Huberta's case, was not a rare complication. We are aware of the circumstances of Huberta's death only through stories that Mama Lily told. No such stories of Sarah's death survived to later generations. However, if Huberta and Sarah shared Lily's internal issues (as I later did), and considering the fact Huberta and Sarah died in their early 40s, and Lily began to suffer from her rectocele in her early 40s, it may be that the women's untimely deaths were due to genetic factors beyond their control. This is especially true in light of the long deliveries of my grandmother, my mother, and later me. As a side note, I have found no other women on any of my other female lines (and I have done extensive genealogical work on all my lines for several generations back) that had women that died as a result of childbirth except for this Kelley and Honeycutt line via the Grays.

Rectoceles result from tears in an area between the rectum and the vagina known at the *rectovaginal septum*. Normally, this is a tough, fibrous wall, but tears, typically through childbirth or a hysterectomy, compromise the integrity of this divider and render it weak enough a tear develops. When this happens, rectal tissue bulges through and into the vagina as a hernia. In its early stages, it is more a nuisance than anything else and may not even cause problems. In its later stages, of which my grandmother suffered, the rectum is actually pushing through the thinned wall, into the vagina, and downward, and the kinking thus creates problems with bowel movements, brings on constipation, and can be extremely uncomfortable.

And, you guessed it, I suffered from a rectocele for pretty close to ten years starting in my early 40s as well. Other females in my family also have eerily similar colon conditions.

In Mama Lily's case, her son Alan Griswold was born weighing thirteen pounds, and as you can probably tell from the picture, she herself was a very tiny woman. No doubt, this contributed to the rectocele in later years. In my case, I had carried and given birth to twins after nearly twenty hours of labor. The birth of both boys was vaginal, but forceps were used on the second child. It has been proven their use further predisposes a woman to a rectocele as well as any number of other conditions. I think it highly likely that Huberta and Sarah, Lily's mother and grandmother, suffered from similar rectoceles which also appeared in their early 40s and which may have well been a complication of pregnancy and childbirth.

In a further mirroring of my great-grandmother, in 2013 at the age of 50, after my third bout with diverticulitis (the second bout exactly two years previous) my colon perforated. After several days and an enormous amount of antibiotics which did not help, it was determined that I needed to have a foot of my colon removed, a temporary colostomy put into place, and a resection done in about three months.

For my great-grandmother, in 1956 there was little they could do in regards to abdominal infections or ruptures.

While it is obvious there is a powerful genetic predisposition to colon issues in the women of my family, some of my issues were also brought on by over-the-counter pain medications I took, sometimes in larger quantities than I should have, in order to control my migraines which were – you got it – inherited from my mother's paternal side of the family through her great-grandmother Anna Lee Whitehead. Later, I was prescribed verapamil for migraine control, and while I experienced some relief with it, I also experienced more frequent bouts with my colon. The problem, for some reason, tamed itself while pregnant with the twins, which I admit was rather odd. To my consternation, however, it mushroomed after their birth.

In actuality, all of these colon issues, at least in my case, were not only driven by genetics, but were tied to and/or exacerbated by a failing thyroid. Constipation is, in fact, one of the more common complaints among hypothyroid sufferers, as the metabolism is not gearing high enough to motivate the colon into moving and thus doing its job.

Needless to say, I knew even as I married in my early 30s that I was a low energy person and working outside the home while having children was going to be problematic. The husband unit attached to me was little better due to what later turned into long-standing and undiagnosed heart issues and his busy job as a registered nurse in the operating room. Nurses may be the only subgroup that, under the right circumstances (or wrong if you choose to be honest) are as overworked as schoolteachers. I will say I never considered working while my children were under school age, for it had always been a given that I would stay home with whatever children we had when they were little. While the husband did not necessarily share the same enthusiasm as I over this decision, it became quite apparent early on that it was simply too cost prohibitive to send two infants to daycare. My concern at this time had been working <u>while</u> the children were older and in school, and by the time the boys <u>were</u> this age, I was not only battling a low-energy body and a need for lots of sleep, but more severe colon issues as well.

Despite my reservations at how well I could handle taking care of my children while working outside the home, I bowed to pressures inside and outside the family and took the job. At least at this time, with some probiotics, a very specialized diet, and stool softeners, my colon issues seemed to be under a moderate amount of control. As for the sleep, how much of it played a role in my early years of thwarting off hypothyroidism, which I believe I had acquired in college or earlier, I do not know. That it played a *major* factor in what happened that second year I worked I have no doubt. A body which needs ten hours, can function adequately on eight, but is only getting four or five and later none at all (as my thyroid began to completely fail), simply is not a body able to fulfill its duty or station in life.

While working I was oftentimes up until 11:00 or so at night grading papers, doing laundry and simple household chores (forget the complicated ones, like baseboards and ceiling fans, and who needs a clean toilet anyhow?). Halfway through the year, I began to notice that even at 11:00 I was not able to fall asleep. Sometimes I would lay awake until 2:00 a.m. At other times, I would fall asleep at 11:00 or 12:00 only to wake up at 3:00 or 4:00 in the morning. What became a need to stay up later became an inability to sleep earlier even had I wanted to. And that later became an inability to sleep at all.

Regardless of when I fell asleep or when I awoke, I had to be up by 5:30 or 6:00. Once up, the boys had to be readied for school (and by this time they were <u>not</u> early risers). Breakfast had to be made and eaten and the dishes at least placed in the sink. I and the boys had to dress. It sounds simple, but as any working mother knows getting ready in the morning is no easy feat. What should take minimal effort and time can seem to take hours, and then it never fails but mother and children rush out the door regardless of what they have done to try and manage otherwise. Needless to say, stress becomes your unwanted and annoying friend.

While the first year started with me somewhat pumped despite my nerves, the second year started out stressful from day one. Personnel issues seemed to plague my working situation, and as the year progressed, and my disease continued to spiral downward, I was left with little to no ability to cope. Student issues did not help either. (Have I said how much I dislike junior high aged children?) By December of that year I was exhausted. Lack of sleep combined with too much stress is never good for anyone. For someone with a weak thyroid, it can be devastating. By December, for the first time in my life, I was experiencing heart palpitations, and a series of visits to dentists and other doctors had revealed my blood pressure was beginning to run high.

I made an appointment with a cardiologist in Houston. I had an echocardiogram, an EKG, and I ran on the treadmill. My heart was good, but he suggested I wear a 24 hour monitor to assess the heart palpitations. The monitor revealed nothing out of the ordinary of course. As the palpitations were intermittent, it was suggested that I not worry over them. I was placed on medication for the high blood pressure.

About this time my monthly cycle took a hit for the first time ever, for I had always been as regular as clockwork except for the month I found out I was pregnant with the twins. (It has always taken a lot to knock that calendar askew.) As a result my blood flow was lasting into two weeks and more, and so I made an appointment with a gynecologist. An exam and bloodwork revealed that I was pre-menopausal, but otherwise there was nothing out of the ordinary to explain my symptoms. (And even as I write this book at the age of 53 I am still having my cycle, so I question that diagnose to be quite frank.) The gynecologist would, if I wanted, prescribe estrogen.

Warning bells rang in my head. If my estrogen levels were not a problem, why would I want to take more? I had read enough by this time to know that estrogen dominance caused certain physical problems, and it seemed counterintuitive to take something I did not need. I declined and more or less fired the first of many doctors.

That spring, the flu hit our area. Now, let me say that I only get the flu about every ten years, and I can tell you *when* I have gotten it in the past: in fifth grade, in ninth grade, my third year of college while at Texas A & M, one year while I was working in 1993, and then this bout in 2005. This was by far the worst, for it morphed into the only case of strep throat I have ever had, and that piggybacked into bronchitis.

It took me weeks to recover, far longer than the other bouts I had before, and with it came what hypothyroid suffers describe as *brain fog.*

I was not Winne-the-Pooh beneath the *little black rain cloud.*

I *was* the *little black rain cloud.*

I initially chalked my less than stellar health state to the after effects of the flu, but eventually I knew there was something more devastating going on than just a long recovery time. All the while, my colon issues spiraled out of control. I was gaining weight and eating little. The heart palpitations continued. A generalized aching set up deep in my joints and bones. My hair began to fall out in clumps. My nails, never strong, were even more splintery and thin.

My allergies, always bad in later February or early March due to a severe allergy to ash trees, reached new heights of torture unbeknownst to anyone in the history of mankind. For the ten years previous to this, my sinuses would swell for several weeks at the first greening of the ash trees. While not too awful in the daytime, the swelling was worse in the evening. At night, I slept not at all. Like clockwork, the misery culminated into a severe sinus infection requiring bucket loads of medications. About the time I was back on my feet, I endured a similar albeit less severe bout in May when pecan trees bloomed.

For years, beginning in my early 20s, I suffered this way through the early part of each spring. While other people were extolling the advent of spring, I wanted winter back. Various medications would work for a time, but inevitably they would always stop giving me relief – Benadryl (which always made me sleepy), Claritin, Zyrtec, and others. In my late 20s and early 30s I was finally prescribed Singulair, and for the first time I managed to get some relief.

This year, however, not even the Singulair was helping me cope, and I was to shortly learn the first two of many lessons.

First, that doctors are oftentimes overrated, and two, that hypothyroidism . . . is never just about hypothyroidism.

THE LITTLE BLACK RAIN CLOUD DRIPS

I'm just floating around over the ground
Wonderin' where I will drip

Winne-the-Pooh

A. A. Milne, *The Many Adventures of Winnie-the-Pooh*

In reality, my adrenal glands were probably not functioning at all by this point. As a matter of fact I believe, due to a working environment at a public school, that they had been taxed in my early 20s and were probably fatigued well before my thyroid ever failed me. Whether it was the adrenals that caused the hypothyroidism, or the other way around, I will never know. One thing was certain by this time, however, and it was a lesson I learned well – the adrenals and the thyroid are intimately linked, and once the adrenals begin to show signs of stress, the thyroid cannot be healed without dealing with the adrenals as well, if not first.

The adrenal glands sit right above the kidneys. They are a little over two inches long and about an inch wide. These glands have two parts: the adrenal cortex and the adrenal medulla. The adrenal cortex is the outer part of the gland and produces hormones that are essential for life. Two such hormones are cortisol and aldosterone. Cortisol helps regulate metabolism and also helps your body respond to stress. Aldosterone, among other things, helps to control blood pressure.

The inner part of the gland, the adrenal medulla, produces hormones that are not necessarily vital to life but do impact the quality of life. One such hormone is adrenaline (yes, that's right). Adrenaline helps your body react to stress, in either a good way, if it is being regulated properly, or bad if not. Adrenaline, as most people know, prepares your body to spring into action in a stressful situation.

When the adrenals begin to muck up the release of hormones and steroids, the result is a condition known as *adrenal fatigue*. There are a number of books and websites that list symptoms of adrenal fatigue (the website Stop the Thyroid Madness is particularly helpful), but for me a few stand out. The first was the appearance of heart palpitations. While mine were probably a combination of low progesterone at the end of my cycle as well as a failing thyroid, no doubt low functioning adrenals did not help the situation. Another was the inability to handle bright lights, especially the sun. Was this due to aging? Perhaps, but not entirely. After all, I was in my mid-40s. That really was not that old.

One of the biggest issues for most people with thyroid related adrenal fatigue is the hormone cortisol. In a person with well-functioning adrenal glands, cortisol levels rise and fall throughout the twenty-four daily cycle. Typically, these levels start to fall in the evening hours, eventually being at their lowest from midnight to about 4 a.m. At that time, they begin to rise and eventually reach their peak again around 8 a.m. in the morning and just in time to get your day started. Any deviation from this, whether due to high cortisol or low cortisol, can interrupt sleep patterns. Since I was not going to sleep till well after 11:00, I had set myself into a vicious but typical cycle due to the whacky cortisol levels.

Cortisol is oftentimes referred to as the stress hormone because it kicks in overdrive when a stressful situation occurs, whether it's an illness of a family member, a financial distress, a sick child, or even a situation perceived to be as dangerous. Because of this it is oftentimes referred to as the *flight or fight* hormone. It is designed to rise intermittently as needed for short-term stress – sort of a burst of energy to deal with whatever situation one is in.

In the case of hypothyroidism, as the thyroid fails the body goes into stress and the adrenals kick in to try and compensate by emitting more cortisol. Rather than the normal rising and falling, cortisol levels remain high and thus the circadian rhythm is thrown out of whack. This results is an inability to fall asleep and/or stay asleep as the adrenals drive the body into a constant *fight or flight* state. This state of high cortisol, combined with little to no sleep and a near constant state of exhaustion, in turn impacts blood sugar, blood pressure, and a whole host of other health related issues.

While disrupted sleep is the most predominant symptom of adrenal fatigue, other common complaints include lack of energy, poor digestion, blood sugar swings, poor decision making abilities, impaired memory, depression, poor sexual function and reduced fertility, and an increase in allergies and infections of one sort or the other. The last is because long standing stress of the adrenals results in an *over reactive* immune system. Notice, I said *over reactive*. This means that your immune system sees everything it comes in contact with as an enemy and battles it accordingly, even to the point of turning on itself (rheumatoid arthritis, lupus, etc.). I often tell people when they complain of allergies that they need to look to the adrenals as the source of their problem.

Mainstream doctors, while recognizing adrenal insufficiency (Addison's disease, Cushing's syndrome), do not acknowledge adrenal fatigue. It does not show up in regular blood work and must be checked either by saliva testing or through a specific, targeted blood test. Neither of these tests, as you have probably guessed by now, are done by regular doctors, so in order to test for adrenal fatigue you will need to seek a wellness or naturopath doctor. And, as with so much of this stuff, you will probably have to pay for it yourself. Insurance is not likely to help.

All of this knowledge, of course, came to me later. What I knew this spring was that I was miserable and my allergies were worse than they had been in years. There appeared to be no relief in sight, and combined with other distressing symptoms, I was getting sicker and sicker.

Besides the run-away allergies, I also lost the ability to multi-task. For a person who could always do multiple things at one time (provided I had enough sleep), it was disturbing to find that I had to focus on one thing at a time.

I would stop loading the dishwasher and turn to face one of the boys, repeating in my head and sometimes with my mouth what they had just told me so I could process the information.

I would reread a sentence in a student's paper several times to understand it, and sometimes I would have to reread parts of/or the whole paper just to be sure and grade it accurately. It did not help that at the time I was an English teacher.

Before this spring I could have loaded the dishwasher while reading a paper and listening to the boys talk all the while planning for the next day. To not be able to do so was upsetting in the least.

When I started playing solitaire at night on the computer when I couldn't sleep simply so I could convince myself that I could still think, I knew there was a problem. Some of this, of course, was due to the lack of sleep, but as any hypothyroid sufferer will tell you, hypothyroidism tiredness and fatigue is **not** the same as being tired from working too hard or not getting enough sleep. It's a whole different kind of fatigue and brain fog. Even at this time I could tell the difference, although I still lacked an explanation.

Another equally frightening symptom that now invaded my world was what hypothyroid sufferers refer to as *air hunger*. I never had asthma (although one child does have asthma), but I would imagine it would have felt somewhat like that. I cannot really say. The best description is as if your lungs cannot quite expand enough to get a full breath of air. I would wait, and then take another, and another. Finally I would get a full breath and then start the process over. I learned early on to at least not panic, for that only made the situation worse, and I knew I would eventually get a whole breath because I always did. For some reason the problem was always worse at night as I tried to fall asleep. With that particular task already at challenge, the air hunger only added to the misery.

Awake at night already, I began to spend long hours researching my symptoms and trying to come up with a reasonable explanation for what was happening to me. In the end, I became convinced the only logical explanation, and the only problem that hit all the symptoms for me, was hypothyroidism.

So I was back at another doctor and another and another. One doctor wanted to do a long series of tests for diabetes. Another wanted to do a hysterectomy. All of them refused to acknowledge that it was my thyroid. My TSH level was fine, as was my estrogen, progesterone, and other hormones.

I was told to slow down.

I was told to prioritize my life.

I was told to exercise, lose some weight, and get rid of stress.

I was offered an anti-depressant to deal with the idea of aging.

It was suggested I take a vacation.

And it became increasingly obvious to me that the average doctor does not know a thing about how the thyroid functions nor its massive importance in how it regulates and drives bodily functions and processes on a daily basis.

About this time I had two close personal calls. The first was while driving on a residential street on my way to see my parents. I leaned sideways to grab something in the front seat. I looked up to find a mailbox right in front of me. Fortunately, and I am still not certain how I did so (have you thanked your guardian angel today?) I veered to the left and avoided what would surely have been a bad collision. I pulled to the side of the road and sat a long time. It was unlike me to make such a poor decision and to have such a close call.

The other incident was nearly as bad. At the time we still had an old electric stove in our house with the rings for burners. I had finished making supper and had turned the burner off. For some reason, I wanted to know if the burner was still on. Rather than looking at the control, I put my hand on the burner. In fact, I was in such a fog that I kept the hand there far too long trying to decide if the burner was still hot, and even after I determined it was I could not react fast enough to pull my hand away. The result was a wound coil impression burned into my palm through at least one layer of skin and maybe two.

Needless to say, for the first time I began to be worried that I would *hurt* the boys, not because I was angry and had no control over my temper, but because I was so unable to concentrate and I seemed to be doing such crazy, dangerous things. This, more than anything of the other symptoms, was particularly frightening for me.

That spring I finally turned in my resignation. I had in reality determined the previous November before I became sick that I was not going to sign on for another year. Not to digress, but I had felt the Lord leading me to bring my boys home after kindergarten, but because of outside pressures and expectations I stayed another year. I would not, however, bow to pressure that spring. Money or not (and it was more *not* than *more* for a variety of reasons), I had to resign and get my life back for I was on a one-way train to an early death, and my little black rain cloud was about to spin itself out through slow drips.

I could see that even if no one else could.

THE BLEEDING OBVIOUS

"Can't we get you on Mastermind, Sybil?
Next contestant Sybil Fawlty from Torquay, special subject the bleeding obvious."

Basil, *Fawlty Towers*

I had by this time observed several things in regards to the functioning of my body, the most important being that while I was tired all the time I was even more so during the back end of my cycle. For me, those days were particularly devastating, and I began to plan my schedule knowing that I was going to be hard pressed to accomplish anything on those days. Since I had for years planned short term events based on when I thought my bowel movements would occur, this was an added burden to say the least.

Late that spring on the advice of a friend I made an appointment with another endocrinologist in Houston. This was the third one I had tried in as many months, but he was highly recommended in the care of not only diabetes, but in regards to fertility issues as well.

By this time my thyroid was so decimated that my TSH was actually showing in my blood work. Additionally, this doctor found that I was suffering from hyperpituitarism.

That's right – the thyroid wasn't working at all, and the pituitary was working too much.

The pituitary is a pea-size gland attached to the base of the brain and composed of three parts: the anterior lobe, the intermediate lobe, and the posterior lobe. The anterior lobe controls and regulates several physiological processes, including stress, growth, reproduction, and most importantly for nursing mothers – lactation. The intermediate lobe produces and secretes melanocyte-stimulating hormone. The posterior pituitary is connected to the hypothalamus.

The pituitary gland itself secretes hormones that help control growth (especially in children), blood pressure, particular purposes of the sex organs, metabolism, some aspects of pregnancy, childbirth, nursing, the kidneys, temperature regulation, pain relief, and . . . the thyroid gland.

That's right, the pituitary, like the adrenal glands, is also intimately married to the thyroid. In my case, since the thyroid gland was no longer providing enough Thyroid Stimulating Hormone, the pituitary had ramped up its messages to the thyroid gland to do its job. The result was an extreme excess of the hormone prolactin which resulted in hyperpituitarism. Normally, this condition is the result of a benign tumor, but not in my case.

I also, near the back end of my cycle, was running out of progesterone. Progesterone is secreted by the corpus luteum after ovulation and during the second half of a woman's menstrual cycle. While instrumental in a woman's menstrual cycle and in pregnancy, it serves other functions as well, particularly in regards to stress and pain relief, and it works closely with the adrenals. When cortisol and adrenaline increase, as in the case of long-term stress, progesterone decreases since it is used to produce cortisol and it perceives its job is not needed. This, of course, results in low progesterone and the result can cause migraines, heavy bleeding during periods, and mood changes (anxiety and/or depression). Of course, this is when a pregnancy is not involved. If a woman is pregnant, low progesterone can cause a wide variety of other symptoms and can even result in miscarriage.

In my case, I was left with dwindling energy and increasing fatigue from the time I ovulated (around day eleven) until the end of my cycle (which was typically 23 days long.) I had no tolerance for pain, and I literally ran from anything that might be stressful.

Or I cried.

Naw - bawled was more like it.

Neither running nor weeping are healthy, but I could not seem to face the fatigue or the pressure of making any decisions or dealing with anything unpleasant. As a number of my symptoms were also caused by adrenal fatigue and hypothyroidism – I was, in a word - a mess. (Note: This doctor did not recognize or mention my adrenal fatigue. This was something I came to on my own later. Shame on him!)

I was prescribed Cabergoline for the hyperpituitarism, but the endocrinologist refused to treat my hypothyroidism. This is standard procedure I do believe, for until the pituitary is tamed it will do little good to try and give your body the thyroid hormones it is lacking. Despite not treating the thyroid, after a few weeks I did begin to feel a bit better. Another trip to the cardiologist revealed nothing out of the ordinary in regards to my heart, not even after wearing the halter again. We took our trip to Canada as planned (although my husband offered to cancel it because I seemed to be so tired all the time), and upon our return I spent the rest of the summer resting. Unfortunately, I seemed to make little progress after my initial small results from the Cabergoline.

That fall the endocrinologist agreed to start me on Levothyroxine for my thyroid. I was elated. Real progress was about to be made.

I was over the moon.

I was going to be healed of this debilitating tiredness.

Or maybe not.

From the first day I took it, I had gastric upset. The burning in my chest was akin to an ulcer. I called the doctor who assured me that could not be the case, so I continued to take it despite my better judgment. The gastric upset continued, and I panicked. What if I was unable to take the very medicine that would make me feel human again? Was I destined to feel this way the rest of my life?

If you have not figured it out by now, Google was becoming my best friend. A quick search revealed others who had experienced the same issue with the Levothyroxine, so I called the pharmacist for confirmation. His answer was quick and to the point. Yes, the Levothyroxine, in fact any medication at all, can cause gastric upset depending on the fillers that are in it. This was the first time I had heard of fillers, but I made a mental note to never forget them again.

I put in another call to the endocrinologist, explained to the nurse yet again my problem and what the pharmacist said, and asked for synthroid. The doctor agreed, although he was reluctant and he let me know it.

Now progress was about to be made.

I was elated.

The moon could not get here fast enough for me to jump over.

I was soon to be shed of the debilitating tiredness which was plaguing by days and nights.

And for a time, I was.

By the time I started the synthroid in the fall of 2006, I was nearly a year into this journey (although again I could argue that I had been spiraling into this disease for years). I was feeling better with the hyperpituitarism under control, and once on the synthroid I began to see some mild improvements in my energy level, the clearing of the brain fog, and in my colon issues. I was sleeping better at night, and I was not falling asleep in the middle of morning prayers with my children. By December of that year I was able to get onto a reasonable schedule in regards to homeschooling my boys. My stamina in the day improved, and I was able to once again multi-task.

I do not remember exactly at what point I began to feel worse again, but I did. It was as if I plateaued for a time, then began to backslide.

Remembering how much better I felt when I first went on the synthroid, I was convinced I simply needed a medication boost, and so I made an appointment with my endocrinologist. Bloodwork was done, and I was certain he would up my medication.

He would not.

He said my levels were fine.

I explained to him that I was tiring once again, and that I was beginning to have some brain fog. I told him of the myriad list of symptoms that were coming back.

He told me *it was just something I would have to learn to live with.*

Doctors, truly, are oftentimes overrated.

They also must take a class in *How to be Cruel to Patients 101.*

I was never so angry in my life. I was only 45 years old. I knew I was too young to feel so lousy. I knew he was not taking me seriously.

I doubted he cared, for somehow I had become a mere number on a blood test. I am certain it was the indoctrination from the class mentioned above.

But far worse, I also realized with devastating clarity that I was . . . heaven forbid . . . turning into my grandmother.

⊤HE PAST IS NOT DEAD

The past is not dead. It isn't even past.

William Faulkner

My maternal grandmother, Robbie Eugene Griswold, suffered for years, possibly her whole life, from a variety of mysterious and debilitating illnesses that seemed to have no common thread or source. An aching neck. Poor energy level. Lack of interest in life. Heavy menstrual periods. Whenever I think of her I see her with her hand on the back of her neck, rocking back and forth, her complaints seemingly genuine in their authenticity. Life for her, I am sad to say, always seemed to involve too much effort and pain.

Born to Charlie Griswold and Lily Gray on 12 March 1920 in Camden, Polk County, Texas, it is not known at what age such complaints began, but she was well into them by the time my mother was a young girl. (Lily herself had some rather unique ailments which are discussed on page 17).

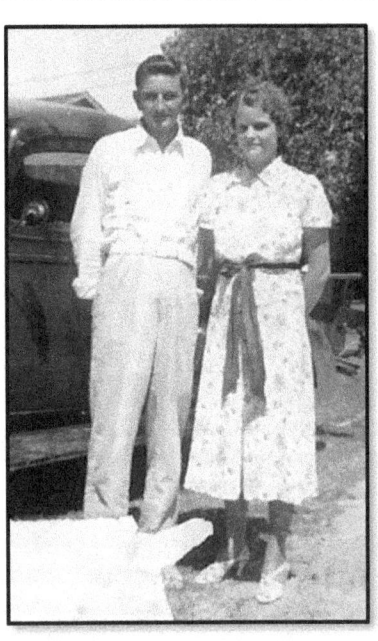

Woodrow McQueen &
Robbie Griswold, about 1837

My mother remembers that for literally *years* my grandmother would have what were called *spells*. These spells oftentimes woke my grandmother in the middle of the night. They were akin to a panic attack, with a racing heart, shaking limbs, and a general feeling of doom. My grandmother refused to stay up alone, and so my mother, being the oldest, was oftentimes the one that had to sit up with her. (My grandfather worked a lot of shift work in those days.) These spells many times landed my grandmother in the emergency room, and at other times she would check herself into the hospital in the hopes that perhaps they could try and find what was wrong. At the time, the word *panic attack* was not in use, but I am certain, and my mother is as well, that this was the cause of my grandmother's suffering.

At some point, my grandmother was placed on thyroid medication, so that my mother remembers that by the time she entered high school my grandmother was interested again in life, she seemed to have more energy, and she seemed to be able to think more clearly. The ER visits stopped as did the hospitalizations.

This lasted several years, but by the time I came along in the early 60s less than ten years later, my grandmother's health had again declined. She was making trips to the ER and the hospital once again, and her spells (panic attacks) had returned, as did her mild yet deepening depression, generalized aches and pains, and her neck complaint. Of course, no amount of x-rays, MRIs, or other diagnostic tools ever found anything wrong in her spine or neck to cause such frets, and the doctors would send her home with the words *nothing is wrong with you.*

The story gets stranger in relation to her fraternal grandmother and my great-great-grandmother. Henrietta Eugenia Durden was born on 27 May 1860 in Alabama. On 30 March 1876 at the age of 16 she married Kinchen Henry Griswold in Butler County, Alabama. By the time the 1880 census was taken, they had moved to Grimes County, Texas, and by 1900 (there is no 1890 census) they were living in Tyler County, Texas. They would remain in this area the rest of their lives. Kinchen died in 1910, and Henrietta, now aged 50, eventually moved in with her son and daughter-in-law Charlie and Lily (Gray) Griswold.

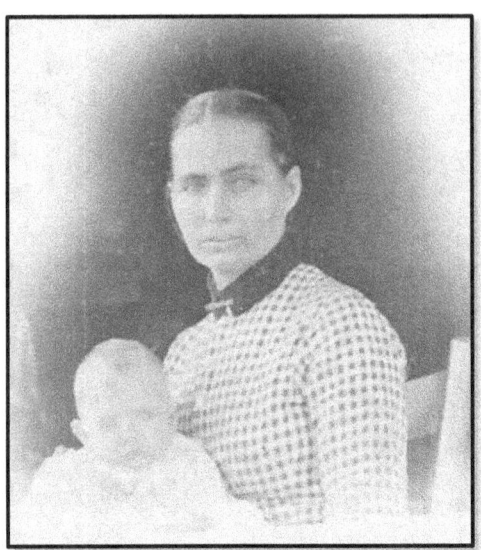

Henrietta Durden Griswold
probably abt 1880

The story I was told was that she pulled her chair up at the age of 50, sat down, and never really moved again except to go to the table and/or to the bed. Most of the time, the story is told that she was lazy, but in light of my now diagnosed condition I began to wonder.

Henrietta suffered in later years from a buffalo hump on her spine. I remember being told when I was growing up that I needed to *straighten my spine* while standing or I would *grow a hump like Grandma Henrietta*. I was also given the impression that perhaps she acquired the hump because she sat so much in her later years. That is not the case, but it was the impression I gained as a young child. The interesting part about her *hump* and subsequent pictures, however, was it appeared she may well have been suffering from acromegaly.

Acromegaly is a result of an overactive pituitary gland, or hyperpituitarism, in this case a result of the excess of GH or growth hormone. If this condition occurs in childhood, it is termed gigantism, and the results are more devastating.

That's right. I had a great-great grandmother that suffered from hyperpituitarism.

As for acromegaly, the initial symptom is the enlargement of the hands and feet. Enlargement of the forehead, jaw, and nose usually follow. Joint pain, thicker skin, a deepening voice, headaches and vision problems are also common. Type 2 diabetes, sleep apnea, and high blood pressure can further complicate matters.

Pictures of Henrietta with her family as a young woman in her 30s reveals a body of normal proportions, with smallish features in her face and a thin figure, even after the birth of her children. Later pictures, however, show enlarged hands, and a protruding jaw and forehead (see page 40). That, combined with the story of the hump and her seeming lack of energy as well as mood swings, points to acromegaly as the cause. My mother does remember

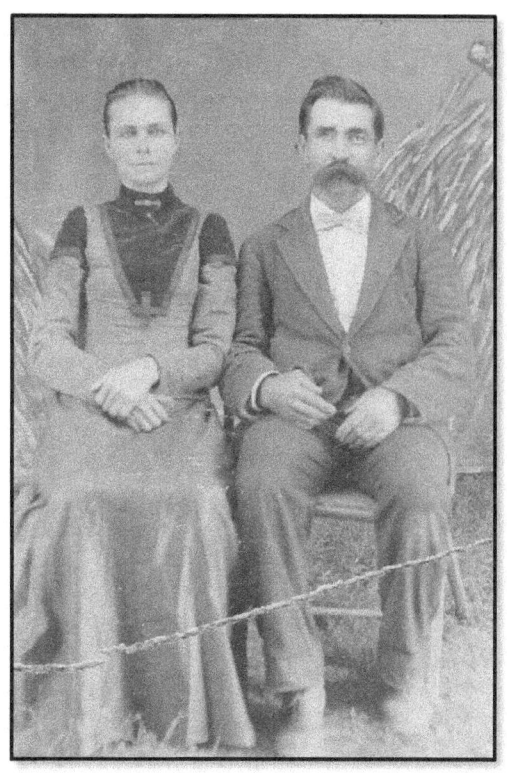

Kinchen Henry Griswold and Henrietta Eugene Durden, about 1895, date based on another picture taken at the same time of the whole family. Notice the size of her hands in proportion to the rest of her body as well as her facial structure.

being told by her aunt that they finally got a diagnosis as to what was wrong with Henrietta, but she could not remember the condition she was told it was she had. She does remember being told the cure was worse than the condition. Likely, it was thought she had a tumor and surgery of such in the 40s and 50s was much different than it would be in today's advanced healthcare system. It must also be noted that it may well have been an assumption at this point that it was a tumor, for there were no sonograms or MRIs at the time, x-rays were limited in their scope, and bloodwork was not easily deciphered or understood.

In 95% of the people diagnosed with acromegaly, the excess growth hormone is due to a benign tumor. That leaves roughly 5% of individuals acquiring the disease through other means, and I do not know at what point in the history of acromegaly it was determined that not all individuals suffering from it had a tumor. Frankly, it is difficult to find much out on this disease at all. It is worthy of note that this ratio is similar to those individuals suffering from hyperpituitarism resulting in an excess of prolactin due to a benign tumor and those that are not.

Acquiring the tumor, of course, is not inherited from parents. Acquiring a weak thyroid or weak pituitary? Perhaps so.

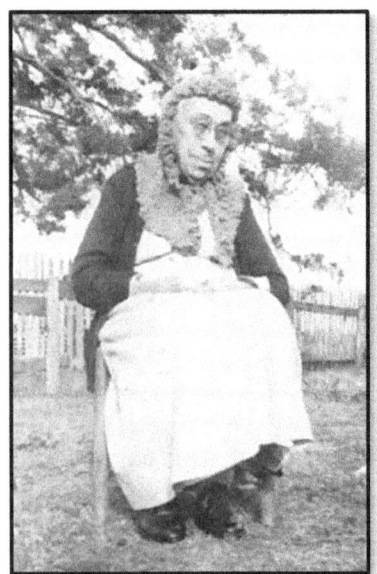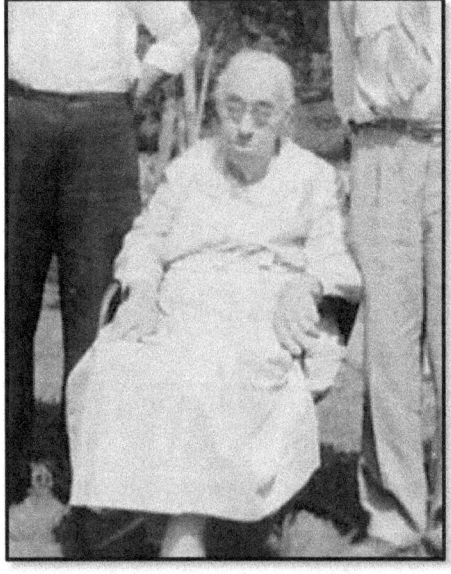

Henrietta Durden Griswold probably about 1950. Notice in the left picture the protruding jaw in relation to the picture of her when younger (see page 37 & 38). In the picture on the right, both the protruding jaw and the enlarged hands in proportion to her head and body are seen.

All of this was, of course, disconcerting. Was there a family connection? Did the women in my family suffer from some genetic abnormality in regards to the thyroid that, when left untreated, ground its way into the pituitary and caused further issues? Did both my grandmother and my great-grandmother suffer from a low to non-functioning thyroid that had never been properly diagnosed but resulted in different and later more severe conditions arising in the pituitary gland? Did my grandmother suffer from hyperpituitarism that was similar to mine in that it affected her prolactin? Did her thyroid become affected as had mine, but she never received a proper diagnosis?

I do not know. I was told by one doctor that hyperpituitarism in regards to prolactin, at least, was not discovered until the early 90s. By then my great-great-grandmother was dead and my grandmother was in the last years of her life. For what it's worth though, I believe in my instance that a large part of my thyroid issues and colon issues are genetic in nature, for my mother has many of the same symptoms as both my grandmother and me. My sister also suffers from a hypothyroid disorder, and I have one son that at one time was nearing a hypothyroid state when he was in junior high as a result of other health issues.

I also believe the pregnancy is a large part of the inducing factor in these hypothyroid issues. I think, based on the timeline my mother gives and the stories of a happy-go-lucky grandmother while in her teens, that her issues came after her pregnancies and births, and each probably sucked her further down into hypothyroidism. My sister has had similar complaints, and while neither my health issues nor my mother's manifested themselves immediately after the birth of our children, nonetheless we can track the beginning of our issues to that time.

With all this anecdotal evidence, it is safe to say that thyroids in my family are weak. And of course, left long enough they affect the pituitary, the adrenals, and other body systems.

Since my endocrinologist refused to acknowledge that perhaps the synthroid was no longer working as it had, it was back to spending time with my best friend Google. What I discovered was unnerving. Although not acknowledged by the mainstream medical community, a large number of individuals who initially feel well on Levothyroxine, whatever its form, later felt unwell.

I was not alone, nor would I be in my fight to find a better drug.

And this new turn of events?

It would completely change the way I viewed healthcare and doctors from this point forward.

It would also, tragically, give me too late a greater understanding of my grandmother.

LOGIC

"Logic!" said the Professor half to himself. "Why don't they teach logic at these schools? There are only three possibilities. Either your sister is telling lies, or she is mad, or she is telling the truth. You know she doesn't tell lies and it is obvious that she is not mad. For the moment then and unless any further evidence turns up, we must assume that she is telling the truth."

The Professor
C. S. Lewis, *The Lion, the Witch, and the Wardrobe*

The first line of defense that most doctors use when a patient has an irregular TSH level is the drug Levothyroxine, also sometimes called L-thyroxine. It comes under a variety of different names, including the most popular name synthroid.

The most important thing for thyroid sufferers to understand is that Levothyroxine is a **synthetic** thyroid hormone **chemically** similar to T4 or the thyroxine that is normally secreted by the follicular cells of the thyroid gland. In other words, it is a man-made compound, and unlike natural desiccated pig thyroid (Armour Thyroid, Nature-Throid), it only contains T4 and <u>not</u> T3.

The use of these man-made compounds first began in the 60s. Before that time, as early as 1891, natural desiccated pig thyroid had been used to treat hypothyroidism. Interestingly, bloodwork, which present day endocrinologists religiously use to determine hypothyroidism and to dose patients by, was not used at the time. Patients were put on the drug **and** dosed according to symptoms.

Natural desiccated pig thyroid is prepared from pig glands. (At one time bovine was also used.) The glands are dried (desiccated), ground to a powder, combined with binder chemicals, and pressed into pills. For those wondering, this was a new use for previously unwanted slaughterhouse offal, and Armour and Company, at the time the largest meatpacker in the United States, was the supplier of the best known brand under the name Armour Thyroid.

The website www.stoptheythyroidmadness.com details the history of desiccated pig thyroid and the maddening twists and turns it has endured due to government regulations beginning in 1906. (Yes, that far back!) I will not go into that here, but I do recommend you read it for your own personal knowledge.

It is important to note that since the 60s and the creation of the synthetic drug Levothyroxine the FDA has waged war on natural desiccated pig thyroid. Big Pharma, with the help of government regulations and erroneous medical studies *that clearly ignore anecdotal evidence and patient feedback*, pushed and pushed the new drug on patients. In fact, I remember reading of women who were taken off the desiccated pig thyroid because the new drugs were touted as safer, only to spiral into health issues fairly quickly. Oftentimes, they were ignored in their request to return to their former drug, although doctors freely dispensed anti-depressants, blood pressure medications, and on and on.

The problem is that the thyroid has to convert T4 to T3 in order for the body to use the T3 for energy. An individual can have T4, but if it is not converted to T3 it does little good. Thus, the reason why so many individuals initially report doing well on Levothyroxine but later plateau. Others report never feeling well on the synthetic drug. Obviously, I was falling into the former category, as I had initially felt well but later not so much. I am probably what is referred to as a *non-converter* by some, although I never bothered to ask. All I know is that I did not do well long-term on just T4, but T4 combined with T3 works **really** well for me just as it does for others.

Why the push for Levothyroxine and the all-out war on natural desiccated pig thyroid? Unfortunately, there is not one dynamic going on here, but a number of them.

The first and foremost, as mentioned above, was probably big Pharma, government regulation, and **money**. Anyone who doesn't think big Pharma is out for their bottom line needs their head examined. They wish to make a profit, not heal people because they are kind-hearted and have a desire to reduce suffering.

Doctors, too, are to blame. They go to medical school, and while they are oftentimes the top of their high school classes and very intelligent, I believe they are generally good at memorizing material to pass a class but not good at solving mysteries. Furthermore, the medical establishment is more likely to give you a medication to control a symptom, another medication to control a side-effect of the first medication and on and on. This merely keeps people sick rather than treats them into good health. After all, healthy people put doctors, hospitals, and drug companies out of business. We can't have that now, can we?

As for doctors, they also listen to the theories put forth by the American Medical Association, big Pharma, and various government agencies that natural desiccated pig thyroid is *dangerous*. According to all of these groups, when using a compounded drug you are trusting a lone person to make that pill correctly and – gasp – they might get it wrong. This is bogus, as even in a synthetic situation someone is creating that drug as well, or they are manning machines that do so. It has also been proven that batch to batch of even Levothyroxine or its equivalent oftentimes varies, sometimes more so than natural desiccated pig thyroid.

There is also a claim that dosing to symptoms is dangerous. I really do not understand this charge. First, going only by bloodwork assumes that everyone needs the same level, and if you have not understood by this time that the thyroid is a complex body organ then I have not done a good job with my words. It has been proven that different people feel better or worse at different levels of TSH, T3 and T4. For me. Unless that T4 rises to at least a number in the middle range, I do not feel well.

Not only that, but the levels in regards to bloodwork have been raised and lowered arbitrarily over the years by physicians and medical boards. Clearly, while they love these numbers and ascribe to them religiously, they are not so clear what they should actually be.

One of the most ridiculous statements is that natural desiccated pig thyroid can cause heart problems. All I know is that a person who cannot move is predisposed to heart disease, so any charge it is dangerous in this regard is ridiculous as far as I am concerned. I do realize that some individuals have issues with heart palpitations while on it, but these cases can be dealt with individually. Also, there is a growing body of research which is currently being ignored by many doctors that hypothyroidism predisposes an individual to heart disease and that those taking natural desiccated pig thyroid actually have lower instances of heart disease and heart attacks. This stands to reason since metabolism is a large factor in not only getting up and moving but in blood pumping through our body and our heart, as well as the cleaning out of cholesterol, etc.

Let me also add that being overmedicated for hypothyroidism results typically in hyperthyroidism, and that is an equally unpleasant state. I have had too much, and you quickly learn that you need to back off of it.

As for doctors, most refuse to listen to patients. Some of this is not entirely their fault. Medical schools teach them to worship and honor blood work. Medical schools oftentimes teach them to treat disease, not fix or eliminate problems that cause the disease. They are oftentimes now constrained by health insurance policies and government health-care programs, not to mention they are generally overworked largely due to those policies and programs. This leaves them little time to learn about patient conditions or the latest research in regards to such. (Although, I will be honest, if you are an endocrinologist, this excuse really is a weak one.) Doctors many times operate under the notion that patients do not know their own bodies, that they cannot read and learn anything medical for themselves, and therefore we are to trust a doctor because *the doctor knows best and by golly he is certainly smarter than the patient.*

That has now, sadly, morphed into *the government knows best* for many individuals. I will say, in defense of doctors, even they are frustrated with this mantra.

You really have to get out of this mindset if you are suffering from a condition like hypothyroidism. Doctors don't have time to learn the intricacies of various body systems, especially something as complicated as the endocrine system (unless, again, they are an endocrinologist – then they *should* obligated to do so but apparently most are no). Most could care less about tracking down a mystery and, as stated above, they do not have the time. And, sad to say, endocrinologists are the **worst**.

More than likely my grandmother was initially given natural desiccated pig thyroid, probably Armout Thyroid. This was the late 50s, and at the time that was still the only form of treatment. She would have more than likely been dosed to her symptoms, and as I stated earlier, my mother even as a young teen noticed an improvement in her mother's mood, temperament, and overall general health.

It appears my grandmother, however, like so many others, had been switched from Armour Thyroid to Levothyroxine when it became available. The results were devastating. She never regained the relief she had for those few years. While keeping her barely alive, she began to suffer a variety of symptoms once again, symptoms that continued to harass her the rest of her life. Had she been of a different temperament she might have complained and eventually found someone who would place her back on the Armour Thyroid. But my grandmother, even when she was feeling well, was of a mild personality and tended to trust doctors. In those days, the internet was not available, and one had to literally *seek* information through magazines and journals.

I also became convinced at this time through my research that the only real and lasting relief I was going to get was through the use of a more natural form of thyroid. My endocrinologist, of course, refused to prescribe it, and so, considering his last devastating statement, I fired him and moved on.

Unfortunately, I kept moving and moving, from one doctor to another. I would go to appointments, explain my history, explain what I had learned about synthroid, then request to be placed on Armour Thyroid. Reactions ranged from mild amusement to wild outrage.

It was dangerous.

It could not be controlled.

It could damage my body.

It could cause heart problems.

I tried to explain my body was already being damaged daily. I could feel myself sliding backwards. That surely it was alright to take something that was more natural and not man-made.

I even agreed to suffer the consequences for such a *bad* decision (cough, cough).

Finally, I got smart and just started asking the receptionist before making an appointment if the endocrinologist would prescribe natural desiccated pig thyroid. I went through every endocrinologist on my insurance plan and a few other types of doctors as well. None of them prescribed anything but levothyroxine or a derivative.

I had for some time been looking into Dr. Hotze's work at his clinic in Houston. I had spoken with a number of individuals who, like me, had poor results with regular physicians in treating their thyroid. I called and spoke with the Hotze clinic nurses on the phone, but the prices were exorbitant (they offered only package deals) and they did not take insurance of any kind.

Along with my research into thyroid issues, I became a consumer of a number of health books on diet and illness. During this time I came across one of Suzanne Somer's books, although I am ashamed to say I do not remember which one. In it she spoke of bioidentical hormone therapies, and she mentioned a doctor north of Houston by the name of Dr. Sakina Davis. Dr. Davis had been a general practitioner who became dissatisfied with the way healthcare forced her to treat patients' symptoms rather than looking for the causes of those symptoms and treating patients into better health. One of her areas of expertise was treating hypothyroidism with the use of bioidentical hormones, aka natural desiccated pig thyroid.

Money was tight, but I knew I could not go back to my other endocrinologist, nor could I continue on the same treatment plan I had been on for the past three and a half years. It was no longer working, and while not on a path to clear death at this point, I was not living my best life possible.

In January of 2010 I called and spoke with a staff member at The Woodlands Wellness & Cosmetic Center, and shortly thereafter I made an appointment.

It was the best decision I ever made, and I oftentimes state to anyone who will listen – Dr. Sakina Davis gave me my life back.

DR. SEUSS ANYONE?

Sometimes the questions are complicated and the answers are simple.

Dr. Seuss

The thyroid is a complicated organ. Much like the engine of a car, it drives our system and gives it the energy to perform a number of tasks. If it is not running properly, other body systems whack out or quit functioning altogether. Again, I am not a doctor, so for the ins and outs of *how* it functions, better sources than I are available.

I can state though that the TSH test used by the vast majority of the medical community, including the doctors I had thus far had the misfortune of dealing with, does not determine thyroid function. It does reveal the level of the thyroid stimulating hormone, but it gives no indication how that is being used. In order to determine how well the thyroid is working, it is imperative to do a full battery of blood work in regards to the thyroid, including checking the free T3 and free T4.

I for one, even with my limited knowledge, grasped this. Why doctors cannot I have not a clue. Why they further persist in stating that the free T3 and free T4 are unimportant I will never know, but I have had more than one doctor tell me this.

In my case, both the free T3 and the free T4 were low, and that despite the fact I had a TSH level clearly in the normal range (which was probably a result of the synthroid). Dr. Davis tapered me off the synthroid and cycled me onto the Armour Thyroid.

Within a matter of weeks, if not earlier, my brain fog had eased and my energy level had improved enough that I was once again walking the block and exercising. Over the next few months my hair started growing back. I could multi-task better than I ever had before, and I could tackle projects and stressful situations with gusto and a plan. I began to lose some of the weight I had gained back the last year or so on the synthroid. The aches and pains in my joints eased and eventually left altogether. My heart palpitations ceased. My nails strengthened. I was going to sleep at night, and I was staying asleep at night. I was awake during the day, and the awful feeling of being constantly tired had left me. I was even able to get off my blood pressure medication.

And remember those devastating seasonal allergies I had suffered with for nearly twenty years? The following spring of 2011 I never even popped a pill of any kind. For the first time in years I was able to enjoy the greening of the trees. It was truly a miracle, and it was then I began to learn the connection between the thyroid and the adrenals.

I did have a minor setback in my overall health the fall of 2013 when my colon ruptured just as my great-grandmother's had. The first part of my two part cautionary tale in that regard is that genetics can be a powerful force. Second, that despite the fact you finally get help for your thyroid, some damage can simply not be undone. While I had a predisposition to colon issues, my slow metabolism which had been an effect of the failing thyroid certainly did not help matters.

I had a foot of my colon removed, and I was given a temporary colostomy. Four months, I had a resection. The recovery time after that was fairly quick, and now, for the first time in years I was free of the debilitating bouts of constipation and frequent bowel movements.

The next spring I published my first novel, *Keeping Secrets*. I continued homeschooling my boys, and later took a stint as coordinator of the teens for that group as well as being the treasurer. The boys activities – piano, church, baseball – kept me busy during this time. About this time I finally convinced my mother to see Dr. Davis as well, and for the first time in decades she began to feel better as a number of life-long symptoms very similar to my grandmother's and mine were finally eased.

Throughout this time I took my Armour Thyroid religiously, and I kept my appointments with Dr. Davis. After six years with her, I was relatively free of thyroid issues. When I had setbacks they were minor and generally involved getting bloodwork done and adjusting my meds. These setbacks were nearly always caused by my being sick (which rarely happens) or overtired simply because life had gotten in the way. Granted, I have never been and will never be the Energizer bunny. The thyroid is a delicate machine and can easily be knocked off balance. However, rest is always the best medicine for thyroid health, and I usually rebounded rather quickly when I forced myself to slow down.

As a matter of fact, over those six years on the Armour Thryoid I rarely gave my thyroid a thought. I never thought of myself as having a disease. I never considered just how badly hypothyroidism can derail a person. However, in the spring of 2016 I was to be dealt a shocking blow through no fault of my own, and I was to be painfully reminded of just how far I had come.

And, unfortunately, how far back I could actually fall.

INTO THE WOODS YET AGAIN

These woods are lovely, dark and deep,
But I have promises to keep,
And miles to go before I sleep,
And miles to go before I sleep.

Robert Frost
Stopping By Woods on a Snowy Evening

In February of 2016 I had a yearly visit with Dr. Davis. While at that visit my blood pressure was also high, so it was back to blood pressure meds for me. This was not totally unexpected, as I had been under an enormous amount of stress since my colon ruptured in 2013. In October of 2014 one son had an emergency appendectomy with a weeklong hospitalization. A year after that, in October of 2015, my husband suffered a heart attack which resulted in a triple bypass and an aortic valve replacement. This was the third hospitalization in three years for my family - all nearly exactly a year apart and all requiring a week or more in the hospital.

In between those hospitalizations my mother was hospitalized several times (one after being taken by life-flight into Hermann Hospital in Houston). In August of 2015, two months previous to my husband's heart attack, my father-in-law passed away after a short illness. My husband took emergency vacation time and flew to Nova Scotia. Flights home for him have been rare, for they involve three flights over a two day period with a one night stay in Halifax, Nova Scotia, both coming and going, and they are extremely expensive. One person alone, depending on airfare at any given time, can cost upwards of $1400 or more.

At the time of my visit with Dr. Davis, the same son that had the emergency appendectomy fourteen months previous was at home recovering from yet another emergency surgery he had undergone in February of 2016 from a testicular torsion.

We were also, as to be expected, struggling financially due to all the medical costs and my husband's time off of work. Short-term disability really is a joke.

So, like I said, the elevated blood pressure was not unexpected.

My thyroid levels were fine, however, and my adrenals were chugging along as well. A mild winter had brought the ash trees to bloom, and still nary a peep from my sinuses had burst forth. I was having some significant pain in my hips that, from time to time, was keeping me awake at night. The left hip, particularly, had bothered me as far back as my late 20s and early 30s, but since my husband's heart attack the previous October they had both been a constant thorn in my side (partial pun intended). Now for some reason, rather than just waking me at night, they hurt during the day after I walked in the evening, after a trip to town, when getting out of the car after a long drive, when getting up from the couch, etc. I would ice them down, particularly the left one, rest them a few days by limiting my walking, get them back to feeling better – only to have them flare up again. I reasoned that somehow, either in sleeping on the hard hospital bed, in walking back and forth into the hospital carrying large burdens, or in standing and perhaps sitting so much in the hospital, I had aggravated them. However, at the time of my visit with Dr. Davis I was dealing with them well enough that I saw no reason to mention them to her.

One of my biggest concerns at this visit was the price of my Armour

Thyroid. Throughout 2015 the manufacturer had continued to raise prices on a drug that was literally keeping me and millions of other thyroid sufferers alive. What once cost me $60 for a three month supply, by the time I got a prescription filled in December of 2015 now cost $195.00 for three months.

Dr. Davis suggested I switch to Nature-Throid which was still natural desiccated pig thyroid but was much cheaper. Rather than nearly $65 a month, this form of natural desiccated thyroid cost about $10. I was ready for the switch and for less strain on my pocketbook. She called the prescription into my local pharmacy, and I was set to go. I picked up my prescription, began taking the dosage, and went on my merry way.

In the meantime, I made an appointment with a general practitioner in order to get back on my high blood pressure medicine. He placed me back on fifty milligrams of Toprol XL.

My hips continued spiraling out of control, and sleep became more and more elusive. I really needed to sleep on my back, but that was **not** happening. With finances still tight, I managed the hip pain the best I could, for while frustrating it was not particularly, at this point anyhow, debilitating. This was, however, about to change.

By the end of March, my sleep declined and my allergies worsened for the first time in years. My hips, which up to this point had been manageable, roared into a pain which was near unbearable. My responsibilities did not help matters. I was readying a book for publication in April (*Metes & Bounds III: John McQueen & Nancy Crews, Children & Grandchildren*). A series of family hospitalizations and ER visits with my parents as well as the boys' homeschool banquet in May kept me busy. Looking back, any shock to my system was going to be too much.

What happened, however, was devastating.

I rolled into mid-May with my parents on the mend, the banquet and book finished, and the realization that I was not only exhausted, but something was not quite right. Brain fog was becoming the order of the day. Not only my hips, but my whole body felt every day when I woke as if it had been beaten beyond recognition. I was generally only sleeping 2 ½ to 3 hours at a time due to the hip pain. If that did not wake me, good old insomnia did. The blood pressure was still proving problematic and was refusing to come down to an acceptable level as well.

I also by mid-May began to crave sugar and carbs, something I had not done in the six years I had been on the Armour Thyroid. This was due to the extreme fatigue and my body trying to find energy any way it could.

My hair began to fall out and my hands began to feel carpal tunnel like symptoms for the first time in nearly twenty-five years. Heart palpitations became my best friend. Sleep became my worst.

In retrospect, I should have realized something was terribly wrong when the sleep went awry. For me, that is the first sign that the thyroid is laboring under difficulties, but I had been so busy, and the hips had been such a part of my lost sleep, that I paid little attention to anything else.

Near the end of May after another night of lying awake until 3 a.m. and beyond, I realized it was time I call the doctor to get my thyroid levels checked. For some reason I never considered that the Nature-Throid might not be working, which probably should have been, out of sheer logic, my first suspicion. Thank goodness I did not, for had I gone into Dr. Davis' office and they checked my levels one of two things would have happened. After a lot of head shaking and comments of *no one else has had this trouble with Nature-Throid* I would have likely been placed back on the more expensive Armour Thyroid, or the Nature-Throid would have been increased to a near dangerous level – as I will shortly explain – and I would have been throw into a hyperthyroid state.

It was time for a prescription refill for the Nature-Throid, so I called it in to the pharmacy and, as I had things to do that day, went on my merry, sluggish way. The day had been particularly exhausting, although I cannot remember what I did. I returned home to find a message from

Dr. Davis's office on my answering machine. My first thought was *how odd*, since they rarely call me between appointments.

They informed me that the pharmacy had just called them to inform them that they had been under medicating me for three months, from the first change of Armour Thyroid to Nature-Throid at the beginning of March. Instead of 162.5 milligrams, I had been receiving 16.25 milligrams.

Basically, I had not been medicated at all, and I was experiencing a total collapse of my thyroid.

The pharmacy, of course, apologized. They admitted they failed to put the decimal in the proper place. I was offered my meds free that month (only after causing a scene in the pharmacy – they probably wanted me out of there) and was given a $25 gift card.

Yep, that's it. An apology and $25. Not much compensation to say the least.

After researching their bungle online, I found out I had little recourse. The State of Texas requires by law that pharmacies inform patients and doctors when an error has been made in dispensing medication. (Some states do not even require this.) However, there was nothing else I could do in regards to the matter.

By June I was taking the proper medication, but it takes up to three months for an individual to stabilize. Depending upon the person, it might even take longer. I spent the month of June mostly on the couch too tired to move, too tired to think, too tired to do anything. My next novel was not being written. I was doing no promotion on my other books. My house was falling apart and dust and all manner of things were piling into the corners.

The aches in my joints continued, with the pain in my hips becoming particularly brutal. Every little symptom I had before roared into life: mild depression, wild allergies, hair loss, continuing uncontrolled high blood pressure, headaches, difficult, prolonged, and missed periods, brittle fingernails, dry skin, weight gain, brain fog, air hunger, and –

worst of all - unrelenting fatigue, the likes of which I had not experienced in the nearly ten years since my initial diagnosis.

It was going to be a long, long summer.

TRANQUILIZER ANYONE?

"Well, don't throw in the towel yet, Agnes, dear. Those tranquilizers may see us through yet."

Clara, *The Long Hot Summer*

Unfortunately, coping with hypothyroidism is not a quick fix. Even after starting on natural desiccated thyroid, it can take several months to notice a significant difference in one's health. Some people report needing up to a year to feel completely normal again. Various factors come into play in this regard, from the levels of the THS, free T3 and free T4, to the amount of damage done already and the other symptoms one has. Reversing most of that is possible, but it takes time, perseverance, and patience.

And no, tranquilizers are not an option, regardless of one's desire for a quick fix.

I had forgotten just how sick I had been before and how quickly one can deteriorate without the proper medication. By June, despite the fact I was back on my full dose of Nature-Throid, the down spiral continued. I managed to wash a few clothes, put some meals on the table, and do a little shopping when absolutely necessary. However, each of those chores wiped me out, and I got little else done otherwise. My blood pressure was still not being controlled well, so it was back to the doctor for me. This time, seeing as how this was my third trip since March, I could see he was getting frustrated. I had intended to discuss my hip pain with him, but he insisted on focusing only on the blood pressure.

He doubled my Toprol XL, bringing it to 50 milligrams twice a day, and then told me to see him in three months.

I was a wittle bitty bit peeved. First, when I mentioned the hip he said I had *bigger problems than that.* He then, however, refused to tell me what the blood pressure reading was, and he further refused to listen when I tried to explain that in coming there that morning I had a number of setbacks, including a flat tire on one vehicle and a last minute switch to another that I had never driven before.

And I was not happy with the plan of treatment. Doubling my Toprol XL but then not wanting to see me for another three months did not seem like good medicine if it was truly that high. At the very least, he should have requested I come back in two or three weeks for a blood pressure check.

As for the hip, he basically said I was getting old and prescribed me an ibuprofen cream rather than sending me for x-rays and/or considering some sort of diagnosis. (I cannot take OTC ibuprofen due to ulcers which I had been diagnosed with just prior to my colon rupturing several years before.) I had read enough by now to know that bursitis (which I strongly suspected) and arthritis (which was becoming a concern to even my husband) need to be treated differently.

Oh, and the cream did not work.

Of an even bigger concern was the fact that when I tried to explain to him that my thyroid was out of whack due to a mix-up in my medication at the pharmacy, and that some of the blood pressure issues were probably related to my being under medicated, he seemed totally uninterested. I had, on previous visits, tried to discuss my thyroid issues with him and how they affected me, but he had brushed me off and not listened then either. He was only concerned at every visit with whether or not Dr. Davis was a *real* doctor (as opposed to being a fake doctor I suppose?) and an endocrinologist, and he insisted again that I send him my latest blood work from her office – *"so I can be sure you are not being overmedicated."*

I had absolutely no intention of giving him anything of the sort. I was not about to argue with him the need for taking 162.5 mg of Nature-Throid, not when I was experiencing the worst down spiral in my health in years from not being properly dosed to begin with.

I went home and decided to see Dr. Davis to determine how much of my issues regarding my blood pressure were related to my thyroid and how much longer I was likely to feel like a walking zombie. At that visit we came up with a plan for getting my blood pressure back under control, and as far as feeling better, she said it would take another month, perhaps two, and she drew some blood to check a few levels.

Most notably? My free T4 was now at 0.9. With a reference range of 0.8 to 1.8, this was considered low normal. This was the same level I had when I first came to see her six years previous.

That's right.

Three months off my meds, and I was in the same shape I had been when I first came to see Dr. Davis and after having been on the synthroid for at least a year and a half. No wonder I was feeling so exhausted and ill all the time. No wonder my hair was still falling out, my skin was dry and cracking, my heart palpitations were worse instead of better, my bones still ached, I was wearing a carpal tunnel brace on my hand again, I wasn't sleeping at night, hives were wreaking havoc with my skin, and my hips felt like they were grinding bone on bone.

To make matters worse, when the bloodwork was taken I had already been on the proper dosage for nearly two months. Who knows how far down my free T4 actually dropped? (And the latest physician who by now I had fired was worried I was being overmedicated? Geesh!)

My liver enzymes were also slightly elevated, which is not unusual in severe hypothyroid patients, but I could not remember a time when my thyroid had ever been so bad as to cause that. A laboring liver can also cause a disruption in sleep at night, so it was a wonder I was sleeping at all. Dr. Davis prescribed a liver cleanse formula to help the liver get back on track.

It took me another month to feel better, and part of the recovery was hampered by my jockeying blood pressure medicines in order to find something that would bring it down. However, about three weeks after my visit to Dr. Davis, a lightbulb came on in my brain. It was as if I was Sleeping Beauty awaking from a long rest. The brain fog cleared and was gone more often than not. My carpal tunnel symptoms improved. The rate at which my hair was falling out slowed. The joint pains eased. My heart palpitations gradually went away.

About this time I finally made a trip to an orthopedic doctor in regards to my hip. I chose to have a shot of cortisone injected into the left hip, and for the first time in nine months I was symptom free and was sleeping again for long stretches at night.

As I write this book, I am four months back on the Nature-Throid. I am having more better days than not. I have managed to write halfway through my next novel and am excited to finally have the voice of my characters back in my head. I have found the energy to write this book, and am planning some book signings at several upcoming fall festivals.

My energy level in the day is almost back to normal, and I am sleeping six to nine hours on an average. In the past month I tackled the messiest house in the world, even rearranging furniture, cleaning out some closets and drawers, and attending things like baseboards and toilets (yea – they do have to be cleaned eventually!). As soon as the weather cools, I intend to hit the yard and especially my flower beds that I neglected this year. Over the summer, I simply did not care. Now, as I walk past them, the deserted, abandoned look of them is bothering me.

There are still nights I awake at 3:00 and cannot go back to sleep. There are days I am still tired and just need to rest. Those days are fewer and further between though.

One thing that becomes more valuable as you near and pass the age of fifty is time. (I heard a priest say this one time, and he was right!) Even one lost day oftentimes hurts, because I will never get that time back. A whole summer lost is maddening. That is perhaps the worst part of this tale and the one I most regret.

Is there anything I can do about it? Not really. Like I said, there is no legal way to hold pharmacies accountable.

Will I still be battling this setback for a while?

I imagine so. I can feel my body has taken a hit. I have had a menstrual flow only once this summer, so this experience may well have thrown me into menopause. I am not certain that I am not experiencing the early stages of rheumatoid arthritis. My allergies are still problematic and the hives are still driving me nuts at times. Due to the hip pain, it is clear I can no longer walk around the block for exercise, so I am looking for another way to stay active. Did the improper dosage make the bursitis worse? I'll never know. I am certain it did not help the situation, especially since there is a strong connection between bursitis and hypothyroidism, just as there is between rheumatoid arthritis and hypothyroidism. All of these conditions are immune related disorders in which the immune system turns on itself, and for some reason these all follow each other in packs.

But with my thyroid levels once again at an optimal level, I am confident I will gradually gain the upper hand on these last symptoms. It will take work, for this is not a disease that is quickly taken care of.

But it is a disease that with proper medication can be managed.

As for me, I can safely say that for now the *little black rain cloud* has left me once again.

I really hope and pray it never comes back.

MIRROR, MIRROR, ON THE WALL

Mirror, mirror, on the wall
Who in this land is the fairest of all?

Little Snow-White
Jacob & Wilhelm Grimm

Looking at ourselves in mirrors is always hard. Looking internally at who we are can be even worse, but oftentimes it is necessary for change. Over the summer (because I was really too tired to do anything else) I had to finally admit to myself that I have a disease. You may well have to admit that at some point in the future, too.

Those of us that are hypothyroid sufferers have days when, even on our meds, we feel tired. There are days when, after having overdone it for several days, we need to rest. There are times, after stressers, that we need to take a break and slow down.

In short, we are not like other people. We have a condition that oftentimes leaves us short on energy and that will require us to take a life-long medication. It is not a health condition that is somewhat of a nuisance, and that by taking the proper medication our quality of life might be somewhat improved. It is a health condition that, if not treated and monitored properly, can morph into and affect our entire health in a number of ways.

Hypothyroid sufferers are prone to rheumatoid arthritis, tendonitis, bursitis, heart disease, fibromyalgia, chronic fatigue syndrome, lupus, and the list goes on and on. If not treated it can lead to death, not from the hypothyroidism itself, but from a secondary cause as a result of the hypothyroidism.

This is probably the single biggest misconception that others have about hypothyroidism. They think it can be cured by eating a better diet. They think you will feel better if you exercise more. They chide you to lose weight, sure that will fix your woes. They suggest more medications, bio-feedback, and yoga. After all, you don't look *too* sick, or perhaps you don't look sick at all.

They simply do not understand how debilitating this disease can be and that such thinking is part of the problem and not part of the cure. Sadly, oftentimes it is those closest to us that have the least patience, and having to explain ourselves or instruct our own families and friends just adds to the stress and madness we are already feeling.

As for my long, hot summer, there were a number of other things besides admitting I had a disease that I came to realize while sitting on the couch too tired to move. I shall pass them on to you in the hopes of sparing you the tortures I have gone through the past few months.

First, never trust a doctor implicitly.

Well yes, I knew this. You probably do too after reading about my journey, and that is if you have not already learned such. However, I had to remind myself of it. I had to remind myself to ask questions and to be a bother. It is a physician's job to explain things. We can never assume they know everything about medicine, because they have proven time and again they do not. If they lose their patience, or refuse to listen to reason or research you have provided for them, then fire them and find another.

Another thing I learned? Never trust your pharmacy. Make sure your dosages are on the up and up. Make sure your pills look the same. Be sure to ask the doctor, if they are calling in a medication or changing it, what the dosage is and the amount at which you should be taking it.

Never take for granted that you are well if you have been diagnosed with hypothyroidism. This is not a disease where you simply take a pill and go on your merry way. You have to sleep and rest. You have to eat a healthy diet. You have to keep stress to a minimum. It can all too easily sneak back up on you, even if you are being medicated properly.

As I stated in my introduction, this was my journey. There are as many journeys with this disease as there are people. My coping mechanisms and skills may not be what works well for others or what they even have at their disposal to use or access. I know of others who have coped in ways other than how I have, but I will say that such treatment *almost always involves the use of natural desiccated pig thyroid.* Frankly, I do not know anyone who has been on Levothyroxine or its equivalent for a number of years who has ever said *I feel great now!*

I encourage you, if you have symptoms similar to mine, or any of the many other symptoms indicative of thyroid disease, to continue seeking a doctor that will help you manage your disease. If you are getting unsatisfactory results, keep looking. If you have to save money and bypass insurance and pay on your own, then do so. You will not regret taking care of your health, but the reality must be faced that you may well have to go outside the medical establishment to get the help you need. If you have learned nothing else from this book, that should come through loud and clear.

If you are on the road to recovery, keep at it. Do not lose hope in small setbacks. This is not a disease to be trifled with. You will have good days and bad days, but eventually the good days should outweigh the bad.

And if you are feeling your best? Then I hope you enjoyed reading about my journey. If you have a similar one, perhaps you too could write it down? If you are not a writer, then feel free to share my story with others. All these words in my head should be good for something.

As for sources that might help you navigate this disease – the website *Stop the Thyroid Madness,* as well as the book by the same name, is the best most up-to-date source I have come across. I encourage you to check it out and to like them on their Facebook page as well. I have read of patients taking the book *Stop the Thyroid Madness* to doctor appointments with portions highlighted in order to try and get some help in regards to their thyroid. Sometimes doctors listen, other times they do not, but that is one strategy for getting the help one needs.

Patient advocate Mary Shomon has a number of books on thyroid issues. She can be found at her website www.verywell.com as well as Facebook. I highly recommend her books especially in regards to *living well* with hypothyroidism. She even has a book on navigating pregnancy if you suffer from this disease.

There are obviously other sources, but these are two of my favorites.

And lastly and most importantly – **you have to be your own best advocate!** No one else knows <u>you</u> like <u>you</u>. No doctor, no matter how genuine, has the investment in your body that you do.

Learn to listen to yourself.

Be good to yourself.

Do whatever you have to do and spend whatever money you have to spend to heal yourself.

After all, we get one body and one life.

We owe it to ourselves and to those we love and who are counting on us to live our best life possible!

A SPECIAL REQUEST

Please, if you enjoyed *Will Someone Please Shoot the Cuckoo?*, would you consider writing a review on Amazon (http://amazon.com/author/donnahechlerporter) and/or Goodreads (http://goodreads.com/donnahechlerporter)? It need not be lengthy, a few words as to why you liked the book will suffice. If you still do not feel comfortable, a rating is always appreciated. Reviews and ratings are a great way for readers to discover new authors, and Donna would very much appreciate any kind words you could write.

ABOUT THE AUTHOR

Donna Hechler Porter graduated from Texas A & M University with a B.S. in Education. After many years of teaching, she now homeschools her twin sons and is active in her local homeschool group. She tutors children in reading, writing, and flute. She has published four genealogy books on her family history and three novels, and her novels have won numerous awards. She is working on her fourth novel.

If you live in southeast Texas and would like Donna to speak to your book club, genealogy or history group, women's club or writer's group, send her an e-mail. She is quite likely to say yes.

You can connect with her via her website http://donnahechlerporterbooks.wordpress.com or by e-mail donnahechlerporterbooks@gmail.com.

AUTHOR LINKS

Donna's Website and Blog *Bringing the Past Into the Present, One Book at a Time* http://donnahechlerporterbooks.wordpress.com.

Donna's Pinterest Page http://pinterest.com/dhporterbooks.com

Donna's email: donnahechlerporterbooks@gmail.com

Donna's Goodreads page:
http://goodreads.com/donnahechlerporter

Follow Donna on

Facebook http://facebook.com/donnahechlerporter.author and

Twitter http://twitter@DHPorterauthor.com.

Follow Donna on Amazon
http://amazon.com/author/donnahechlerporter and you will receive emails concerning new releases.

Sign up for Donna's quarterly newsletter
http://madmimi.com/signup/136827/join.

Family members can also find Donna on her genealogy blog *The Flying Shuttle* http://theflyingshuttle.com/blogspot.com and descendants of John McQueen and Nancy Crews can connect with her on Facebook on the *Descendants of John McQueen & Nancy Crews* Facebook page
https://www.facebook.com/groups/1548695412018847/).

www.ingramcontent.com/pod-product-compliance
Lightning Source LLC
Chambersburg PA
CBHW070125290526
45789CB00005B/2144